Super Blueberries

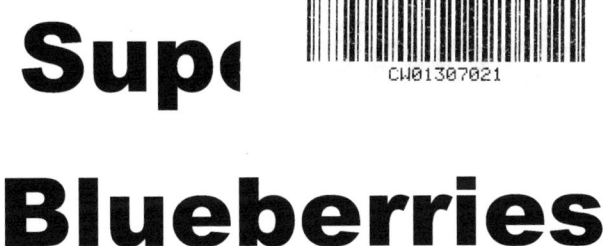

Quick and Easy Blueberry Recipes for Healthy Living

Sarah Spencer

Copyrights

All rights reserved © Sarah Spencer and The Cookbook Publisher. No part of this publication or the information in it may be quoted from or reproduced in any form by means such as printing, scanning, photocopying, or otherwise without prior written permission of the copyright holder.

Disclaimer and Terms of Use

Effort has been made to ensure that the information in this book is accurate and complete. However, the author and the publisher do not warrant the accuracy of the information, text, and graphics contained within the book due to the rapidly changing nature of science, research, known and unknown facts, and internet. The author and the publisher do not hold any responsibility for errors, omissions, or contrary interpretation of the subject matter herein. This book is presented solely for motivational and informational purposes only.

The recipes provided in this book are for informational purposes only and are not intended to provide dietary advice. A medical practitioner should be consulted before making any changes in diet. Additionally, recipe cooking times may require adjustment depending on age and quality of appliances. Readers are strongly urged to take all precautions to ensure ingredients are fully cooked in order to avoid the dangers of foodborne illnesses. The recipes and suggestions provided in this book are solely the opinion of the author. The author and publisher do not take any responsibility for any consequences that may result due to following the instructions provided in this book.

ISBN: 978-1537656205

Printed in the United States

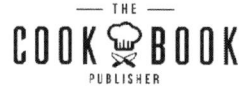

Avant-Propos

Blueberries might be small in size but they certainly punch above their weight in the health department. Blueberries are an excellent source of vitamin C and manganese, which aids in the development of tissue growth as well as in processing cholesterol and nutrients. They are also low in fat and high in dietary fiber to make you feel fuller faster and aid in weight loss.

Blueberries' signature dark blue skin is rich in antioxidants, which are said to have age-defying properties and which are necessary for the normal functioning of our immune system, skin health, and overall bodily functions. Ongoing studies suggest that these berries are anti-inflammatory and might reduce the risk of heart disease, cancer, and a host of other chronic illnesses.

Loaded with health benefits, blueberries are delicious on their own. They are sweet and tangy and appealing to people of all ages. This makes it easy to introduce them to even your fussy kids, by throwing a handful into breakfast bowls or salad lunches.

As a cooking ingredient, blueberries emit a beautiful deep bluish-purple hue that gives dishes like pies and cheesecakes their signature color. When cooked, they release plenty of juices to moisten sweet and savory dishes, and also give a fresh, earthy flavor to jams, sauces, and relishes.

This book presents 50 recipes that use fresh, frozen, or dried blueberries to boost your nutrition intake of this superfood. Sneak these blue beauties into muffins or cupcakes, or perhaps try out some more unconventional ways to eat them, like scattering them onto pizzas, or putting them in burgers.

Start flipping through this cookbook and explore some fun ways to use blueberries for your next recipe!

Contents

Introduction 1
   Choosing and Storing 2
   Baking with Blueberries 3
Breakfast Recipes 5
   Blueberry Smoothie Bowl 5
   Blueberry Quinoa Breakfast Bowl...6
   No-bake Blueberry Breakfast Bars 7
   Blueberry and Almond Granola..9
   Lemon Blueberry Pancakes...11
   Blueberry and Banana Bread 13
   Yogurt Cups with Blueberry Compote...15
   Blueberry Bagels 17
   Baked Blueberry French Toast...19
   Blueberry Belgian Waffles 21
Savory Recipes 23
   Fresh Watermelon and Blueberry Salad...23
   Wild Rice Salad with Corn and Blueberries 25
   Vegetable Couscous with Blueberries 27
   Blueberry and Caramelized Onion Pizza 29
   Mushroom and Blueberry Balsamic Pot Roast.................................31
   Flank Steak with Blueberry Sauce 33
   Juicy Blueberry Beef Burger 35
   Grilled Chicken with Blueberry Guacamole 37
   Pork Chops with Tangy Blueberry Sauce 39
   Broiled Salmon with Blueberry Glaze...41
Appetizers and Snack Recipes 43
   Blueberry Banana Muffins 43
   Peach and Blueberry Salsa with Brie 45
   Blueberry Buttermilk Scones 47
   Blueberry and Lemon Squares..49
   Yogurt-Coated Blueberry Bites 50
   Blueberry Frozen Yogurt Ice Cream 51
   Almond Blueberry Oat Bites..53
   Blueberry Sunflower Energy Balls 55
   Chewy Blueberry Gummies 56
   Blueberry Coconut Bars 57

Dessert Recipes 59
  Baked Cheesecake with Blueberry Compote...................59
  Classic Blueberry Pie 62
  Blueberry Bread Pudding 65
  Blueberry Coffee Cake 67
  Blueberry and Buttermilk Tart 69
  Blueberry Ice Pops 71
  Blueberry Swirl Cupcakes 72
  Blueberry Cobbler 75
  Lemon Blueberry Pound Cake 77
  Blackberry and Blueberry Turnovers 79
Drink Recipes 81
  Blueberry Ice Lemon Tea 81
  Chocolate Blueberry Smoothie 83
  Blueberry Pineapple Mojito 84
  Blueberry Ginger Bellini 85
  Red Wine Blueberry and Peach Sangria 86
Condiment, Dressing, and Sauce Recipes 87
  Blueberry Chia Seed Jam 87
  Blueberry Chipotle Chutney 89
  Blueberry Cheddar Dip..90
  Blueberry Dessert Sauce 91
  Blueberry Vinaigrette 92
Conclusion...93
About the Author..95
  More Books from Sarah Spencer 97
Appendix - Cooking Conversion Charts 101

Introduction

Blueberries have now become a staple in the fruit aisle of many supermarkets and grocery stores. Originally from North America, they are now grown all over the world. Fresh blueberries are typically most abundant throughout the summer, though frozen varieties are available all-year round.

Given its ubiquity, it is easy to forget that this tiny blue fruit is the granddaddy of the superfood trend. Multiple researches have shown that these berries generate a host of short-term and potentially long-term health benefits.

Blueberries are a good source of dietary fiber, and vitamins C and E. Sweet and juicy, they are a natural and healthier alternative to candies and sweets for days when the body craves sugar. At 84 calories per cup, blueberries are low in calories and make you full faster, which makes them ideal for weight loss purposes.

High levels of flavonoid make blueberries one of the best sources of antioxidants. Antioxidants have not only been associated anti-aging properties, they also protect our bodies against stress, cancer, and arthritis, among other diseases. Small-scale studies show that blueberry consumption slows down mental aging, and stimulates the growth of new brain cells. The fruit is said to reduce the inflammation that drives many chronic illnesses, and they strengthen the heart and lower blood pressure.

Given their health benefits, blueberries ought to be a regular item in your diet. They are most commonly eaten raw or thrown into breakfast cereal or yogurt. This cookbook seeks to expand the number of ways of incorporating this superfood into your diet.

Blueberries have a fruity and tart flavor profile, which makes them perfect for adding into sweet desserts, condiments, and baked goods. Likewise, their acidity also makes them excellent for cutting through or acting as an accompaniment to rich and oily cuts of meat, such as lamb, steak, and salmon. Some recipes in this book will provide suggestions for both sweet and savory dishes that will take your taste palette out of its comfort zone.

From the classic blueberry pie to a blueberry, feta, and caramelized onion pizza, there are plenty of ideas for your main meal as well as a variety of desserts, snacks, and drinks that are sure to delight adults and kids alike. There are also tips, tricks, and ideas for choosing and storing this blue dynamo at home, so start flipping the pages to get inspired!

Choosing and Storing

For fresh blueberries, buy those that appear firm and have a slightly silvery sheen. Size does not matter as much when selecting berries, but the color is key to indicating its maturity. Unripe berries are usually green or red near the stem and will not ripen once they are plucked. Choose those that are deep blue or purple in color, and in fact, the darker they are, the more antioxidants they contain. Discard those that have turned soft, are shriveled, or show signs of mold.

To store your blueberries, place them loosely in a covered container and store them in the refrigerator. Keep them as dry as possible because excess moisture will cause them to spoil easily. Only wash the blueberries when you are about to consume them. To freeze fresh blueberries, give them a quick rinse and pat them dry with a tea towel or paper napkins. Transfer the blueberries to a freezer-safe container or a resealable plastic bag and place them flat in the freezer so the blueberries will freeze individually.

Frozen blueberries are also convenient options to reach for in the frozen section of the supermarket. They are as nutritious as the fresh ones because most of them have been flash frozen once picked, so as to lock in their nutrients. When you pick up a bag of frozen blueberries, try to feel whether the blueberries are loose inside the package, rather than in a clump.

Store frozen blueberries in the freezer immediately, and put them away as soon as you are done using them. Defrosted frozen blueberries should be stored in a refrigerator and used within three days of thawing.

Baking with Blueberries

When it comes to baking, there is often an option to choose between using fresh or frozen blueberries. Do note that the frozen varieties tend to bleed more into the batter than their fresh counterpart, which might affect the overall aesthetics of the final product. If you do want your baked goods to feature the prized golden brown hue, you might want to consider using fresh blueberries.

That said, the frozen option is always cheaper – particularly during the off-season months. If you only have frozen blueberries at hand, run them under cold water briefly, until the water runs clearer. Transfer the blueberries to several layers of paper towel and gently pat them until most of the colored water is absorbed. Fold them gently into the batter with as few strokes as possible to minimize the staining.

Another common baking problem is the dreaded sight of blueberries sinking to the bottom of the pan, which creates a mushy mess. This is because the blueberries tend to be denser than the batter, which results in them concentrating at the base.

To avoid this situation, coat the blueberries with a dusting of the recipe's dry ingredients, which helps the berries cling to the batter and spread more evenly throughout. At the same time, the dry ingredients will also help soak up any excess bleeding from the frozen blueberries. Alternatively, spread a layer of batter on the bottom of the pan before adding a layer of blueberries, followed by the rest of the batter and the remaining blueberries. By alternating these layers, you are manually distributing the blueberries throughout the batter without over mixing it, which might cause bleeding.

Breakfast Recipes

Blueberry Smoothie Bowl

Servings: 2

Ingredients
1 cup frozen blueberries
¾ cup almond milk
1 medium banana, sliced
6 strawberries, hulled and sliced
1 tablespoon goji berries
1 tablespoon oats
1 tablespoon hemp hearts
2 tablespoons chia seeds

Preparation
1. In a blender, combine the frozen blueberries with the almond milk until smooth. Transfer the mixture to 2 bowls.
2. Scatter the rest of the ingredients on top of each bowl. Serve immediately.

Nutritional Facts (303 g per single serving)
Calories 265
Fats 10 g
Carbs 41 g
Protein 8 g
Sodium 84 mg

Blueberry Quinoa Breakfast Bowl

Servings: 4

Ingredients
2 cups unsweetened almond milk
1 cup quinoa, rinsed
2 cups blueberries
½ cup chopped pecans
¼ teaspoon ground ginger
¼ teaspoon ground nutmeg
2 tablespoons maple syrup

Preparation
1. In a medium saucepan, bring the almond milk and quinoa to a boil. Reduce the heat to low and continue simmering for about 15-20 minutes, or until most of the liquid is absorbed. Cover the pot and let it sit for another 5 minutes. Fluff the quinoa with a fork.
2. Stir in the blueberries, pecans, ginger, nutmeg, and maple syrup.
3. Best served warm

Nutritional Facts (250 g per single serving)
Calories 425
Fats 21 g
Carbs 52 g
Protein 12 g
Sodium 97 mg

No-bake Blueberry Breakfast Bars

Servings: 16

Ingredients
1 ½ cups rolled oats
¾ cup whole almonds
½ cup dried blueberries
½ cup pistachios
½ cup ground flaxseed
⅓ cup walnuts
⅓ cup pumpkin seeds
¼ cup sunflower seeds
⅓ cup maple syrup
¼ cup unsweetened applesauce
1 cup almond butter

Preparation
1. Line an 8x8 baking pan with parchment paper.
2. In a large mixing bowl, whisk the dry ingredients together.
3. In a small mixing bowl, combine the maple syrup, applesauce, and almond butter. Pour the mixture over the dry ingredients, and stir to ensure that everything is well combined.
4. Transfer the mixture into the prepared pan and press it down with slightly damp hands.
5. Place the pan into the freezer for about an hour.
6. Remove the pan from the freezer. Lift the block out of the pan and peel the parchment paper away. Cut the block into 16 bars. Devour them immediately, or store them inside a sealed bag in the freezer.

Nutritional Facts (67 g per single serving)
Calories 311
Fats 21 g
Carbs 26 g
Protein 11 g
Sodium 4 mg

Blueberry and Almond Granola

Makes: 3 cups

Ingredients
2 cups puffed rice cereal
1 ½ cups rolled oats
1 teaspoon coconut oil, melted
½ cup almond milk
3 tablespoons maple syrup
⅓ cup dried blueberries

Preparation
1. Preheat the oven to 350°F. Line a 9-inch square pan with parchment paper.
2. In a large bowl, mix the rice cereal and oats. In a separate bowl, whisk together the coconut oil, almond milk, and maple syrup. Combine the wet ingredients with the dry ingredients, stirring to ensure that everything is well coated.
3. Transfer the cereal to the prepared baking pan and spread it out evenly.
4. Bake for about 40-45 minutes, taking it out every 15 minutes to give the granola mixture a good stir. Keep a close watch, because it burns easily.
5. Remove the pan from the oven and allow it to cool down completely. The granola will crisp up as it cools down.
6. Stir in the dried blueberries, and it is ready to be served.

Nutritional Facts (170 g per single cup serving)
Calories 456
Fats 6 g
Carbs 88 g
Protein 16 g
Sodium 36 mg

Lemon Blueberry Pancakes

Servings: 4

Ingredients
1 ½ cups cake flour
¼ teaspoon salt
1 tablespoon baking powder
3 tablespoons sugar
1 ½ cups evaporated milk
Juice and zest of 1 lemon
1 large egg
1 ½ teaspoon vanilla extract
2 tablespoons butter, melted, plus more for frying
1 cup fresh blueberries
Toppings: Butter, maple syrup, blueberries

Preparation
1. In a medium bowl, whisk together the flour, salt, baking powder, and sugar
2. In a separate bowl, stir together the evaporated milk, and the juice and zest of the lemon. Allow the mixture to sit for 5 minutes. Mix in the egg, vanilla extract and butter.
3. Combine the wet ingredients with the dry ingredients until just combined. Add the blueberries and fold them in gently.
4. Heat some butter in a large skillet over medium-low heat. Pour the pancake batter into the skillet and cook for 2-4 minutes on each side, or until bubbles appear in the pancake and the bottom is golden brown.
5. Serve warm with more butter, maple syrup, and fresh blueberries

Nutritional Facts (216 g per single serving)
Calories 443
Fats 15 g
Carbs 66 g
Protein 13 g
Sodium 269 mg

Blueberry and Banana Bread

Servings: 1

Ingredients
1 ½ cups all-purpose flour
1 teaspoon baking soda
1 teaspoon salt
½ teaspoon baking powder
½ teaspoon ground cinnamon
½ teaspoon ground nutmeg
1 cup sugar
½ cup vegetable oil
2 large eggs, beaten
2 teaspoons vanilla extract
2 ripe bananas, mashed
1 cup fresh blueberries
Butter, for greasing

Preparation
1. Preheat the oven to 350°F. Grease a 9x5 loaf pan with butter.
2. In a medium bowl, whisk together the flour, baking soda, salt, baking powder, cinnamon, and nutmeg.
3. In a large bowl, beat the sugar, oil, eggs, and vanilla extract. Combine the dry ingredients with the wet ingredients and mix until there are no large lumps.
4. Stir in the mashed bananas and blueberries.
5. Transfer the batter into the prepared loaf pan. Bake for about an hour, or until a skewer comes out clean when inserted into the thickest part of the bread.

6. Remove the bread from the oven and let it cool in the pan for 15 minutes. Run a knife around the edges of the pan to release the bread. Let the bread cool completely on a wire rack before cutting it into slices.

Nutritional Facts (995 g per single serving)
Calories 2838
Fats 123 g
Carbs 420 g
Protein 35 g
Sodium 3737 mg

Yogurt Cups with Blueberry Compote

Servings: 4

Ingredients
2 cups fresh or frozen blueberries
½ cup + 2 tablespoons water
Zest of 1 lemon
1 teaspoon ground cinnamon
½ teaspoon ground ginger
2 teaspoons cornstarch
1 teaspoon vanilla extract
4 cups plain, low-fat Greek yogurt
¼ cup chopped almonds
4 tablespoons honey or maple syrup

Preparation
1. In a small saucepan, combine the blueberries, ½ cup of water, lemon zest, cinnamon, and ginger. Bring the mixture to a boil, then reduce the heat to medium low and continue simmering until all the blueberries have burst, about 20 minutes.
2. Meanwhile, dissolve the cornstarch in 2 tablespoons of water. Pour the cornstarch slurry into the blueberry mixture, together with the vanilla extract. Continue to stir until the compote thickens. Allow it to cool slightly.
3. Scoop the yogurt into 4 serving cups. Divide the blueberry compote evenly among the cups. Scatter the chopped almonds and honey all over the top.

Nutritional Facts (386 g per single serving)
Calories 342
Fats 9 g
Carbs 38 g
Protein 30 g
Sodium 101 mg

Blueberry Bagels

Servings: 8

Ingredients
1 package active dry yeast
2 tablespoons sugar
1 ¼ cups warm water, divided
3 ½ cups + ¼ cup all-purpose flour
1 ½ teaspoons salt
1 cup blueberries

Preparation
1. In a small bowl, scatter the yeast and sugar over ½ a cup of warm water. Set it aside for 5 minutes to activate the yeast. Small bubbles should start forming on the water's surface.
2. In a stand mixer, combine 3 ½ cups flour, salt, the yeast mixture, and the rest of the water.
3. In a small bowl, toss the blueberries in ¼ cup of flour. Fold the blueberries into the dough.
4. Using a dough hook, beat the ingredients together until the dough does not stick to the side of the bowl. It should be soft, elastic, and purple in color.
5. Transfer the dough to a large, clean bowl. Cover it with a dish towel and set it aside in a warm spot for it to rise to double its size, about 1 ½ hours.
6. Punch the risen dough down and transfer it to a lightly floured surface. Knead the dough a few times before dividing it into 8 portions. Roll the dough out into a baton shape and seal the ends to form a bagel. Transfer the bagel to a large baking sheet. Repeat the process until you get 8

bagels. Cover with a dish towel and allow it to rest for another 30 minutes.
7. In the last 10 minutes of proofing, preheat the oven to 425°F, and bring a large pot of water to a rolling boil.
8. Cook the bagels in the boiling water for 3-4 minutes, making sure to turn them over to cook on both sides. Using a slotted spoon, remove the bagels from the water and return them to the baking sheet.
9. Bake the bagels for 20 minutes, or until they are golden brown.

Nutritional Facts (82 g per single serving)
Calories 239
Fats 1 g
Carbs 51 g
Protein 7 g
Sodium 438 mg

Baked Blueberry French Toast

Servings: 8

Ingredients
12 slices day-old white bread, crusts removed
2 (8 ounce) packages cream cheese, cubed
1 cup fresh or frozen blueberries
12 large eggs, beaten
2 cups 2% milk
⅓ cup maple syrup

Sauce:
1 cup sugar
1 cup water
2 tablespoons cornstarch
1 cup fresh or frozen blueberries
1 tablespoon butter

Preparation
1. Start the preparation the night before. Cut the bread into 1-inch cubes, and place half in a 13x9 baking dish.
2. Scatter cream cheese cubes and blueberries over the bread. Finish with the rest of the bread cubes.
3. In a medium mixing bowl, beat the eggs, and mix in the milk and maple syrup. Pour it evenly over the bread, cover with aluminum foil, and refrigerate overnight.
4. The next day, take the dish out of the fridge 30 minutes before baking. Preheat the oven to 350°F.

5. Bake, still covered with foil, for 30 minutes. Remove the foil and bake uncovered for another 30 minutes, or until the eggs are set and the top is brown. Remove the pan from the oven and allow it to cool slightly.
6. To make the sauce, mix the sugar, water, and cornstarch in a small saucepan. Bring the sauce to a boil over medium heat, making sure to stir frequently, until it becomes smooth and has thickened. Add the blueberries and bring it back to a boil. Lower the heat to low, and simmer for another 8-10 minutes, until the berries have burst. Remove the pot from the heat and stir in the butter.
7. Serve the French toast warm with a generous serving of blueberry sauce.

Nutritional Facts (344 g per single serving)
Calories 610
Fats 31 g
Carbs 67 g
Protein 20 g
Sodium 517 mg

Blueberry Belgian Waffles

Servings: 4

Ingredients
2 cups all-purpose flour
1 tablespoon sugar
1 tablespoon baking powder
¼ teaspoon salt
1 ¾ cups milk
2 large eggs
2 tablespoons vegetable oil + more for greasing
½ cup fresh or frozen blueberries
Toppings: Butter, maple syrup, or whipped cream

Preparation
1. In a large bowl, whisk together the flour, sugar, baking powder, and salt. In a separate medium bowl, stir together the milk, eggs, and oil.
2. Add the wet ingredients to the dry ingredients and mix until just combined. Fold in the blueberries.
3. Preheat the waffle iron, and lightly grease it with oil. Pour 1 cup of the batter into the center of the iron grid (adjust the amount if necessary. according to the size of your waffle iron), and cook it until it turns golden brown. Repeat until all the batter is used.
4. Serve the waffles with butter, maple syrup, whipped cream, or any desired toppings.

Nutritional Facts (229 g per single serving)
Calories 414
Fats 14 g
Carbs 61 g
Protein 13 g
Sodium 232 mg

Savory Recipes

Fresh Watermelon and Blueberry Salad

Servings: 6

Ingredients
1 large seedless watermelon
⅔ cup arugula
⅔ cup blueberries
½ cup feta cheese, cubed
3 tablespoons pumpkin seeds
¼ cup fresh mint leaves, finely chopped

Dressing:
3 tablespoons extra virgin olive oil
2 tablespoons red wine vinegar
1 teaspoon Dijon mustard
1 teaspoon honey
Salt and pepper, to taste

Preparation
1. Cut the watermelon in half. Using a sharp knife, run it around the outside of the flesh of the melon, to separate it from the rind. Score the flesh to create a crisscross pattern. Using a large serving spoon, remove the watermelon from the rind. Cut the larger chunks of watermelon into smaller, bite-sized pieces. Transfer the watermelon to a large bowl.
2. Add the arugula, blueberries, feta, and pumpkin seeds to the watermelon.

3. In a small bowl, whisk together all the dressing ingredients, together with any excess watermelon juice.
4. Toss the dressing with the salad.
5. Garnish with chopped mint leaves, and serve.

Nutritional Facts (802 g per single serving)
Calories 361
Fats 13 g
Carbs 61 g
Protein 8 g
Sodium 17 mg

Wild Rice Salad with Corn and Blueberries

Servings: 4

Ingredients
3 cups water, divided
½ cup long-grain brown rice
½ cup wild rice
¼ cup toasted almonds, roughly chopped
1 ear of corn, kernels only
¼ cup dried blueberries
2 tablespoons chopped red onion
Salt and pepper, to taste
2 sprigs parsley, finely chopped

Dressing:
½ clove garlic, finely grated
4 teaspoons fresh lemon juice
2 teaspoons white wine vinegar
1 teaspoon sugar
¼ teaspoon paprika
¼ cup olive oil
Salt and pepper, to taste

Preparation

1. In a small saucepan, bring 1 cup of water to a boil over medium-high heat. Once the water is boiling, add the brown rice and simmer, covered, over medium-low heat for 10 minutes. Remove the pot from the heat. Use a fork to give the rice a stir and prevent it from sticking to the bottom. The rice should still be slightly sticky at this point. Cover the pot and allow the rice to continue steaming for the next 10 minutes.
2. At the same time, bring the wild rice and 2 cups of water to a boil over medium-high heat. Reduce the heat to low, cover, and simmer for another 30-45 minutes. Check that the grains are tender. Remove the pot from the heat and allow it to sit, covered, for 5 minutes. Strain off any excess liquid.
3. In a small bowl, whisk together all the dressing ingredients.
4. Combine both types of rice in a large mixing bowl. Add the almonds, corn, blueberries, and onion. Drizzle the dressing over the ingredients and give it a good toss. Season with salt and pepper.
5. Finish it off with chopped parsley.

Nutritional Facts (217 g per single serving)
Calories 378
Fats 18 g
Carbs 51 g
Protein 17g
Sodium 12 mg

Vegetable Couscous with Blueberries

Servings: 2

Ingredients
1 cup vegetable broth
1 cup couscous
Pinch ground cumin
3 tablespoons olive oil, divided
2 carrots, diced
1 small zucchini, diced
½ cup chickpeas, cooked or canned
Salt and pepper, to taste
¼ cup walnuts, chopped
1 ¼ cups frozen blueberries
4 sprigs fresh cilantro, chopped
4 sprigs fresh flat leaf parsley, chopped

Preparation
1. In a small saucepan, bring the vegetable broth to a boil over medium-high heat. Remove the pot from the burner. Stir in the couscous, pinch of cumin, and 2 tablespoons of the oil. Cover the pot and allow it to stand for 5 minutes. Fluff the couscous with a fork and transfer it to a large bowl.
2. In a medium skillet, heat the remaining tablespoon of oil. Sauté the carrots until they are tender, about 5 minutes. Add the zucchini and chickpeas, and cook for another 3 minutes. Season with salt and pepper. Transfer the vegetables into the bowl with the couscous.

3. Add the walnuts, blueberries, cilantro, and parsley to the bowl. Give it a good toss, and season according to your taste. Serve immediately.

Nutritional Facts (487 g per single serving)
Calories 728
Fats 28 g
Carbs 102 g
Protein 19 g
Sodium 387 mg

Blueberry and Caramelized Onion Pizza

Servings: 2

Ingredients
2 flatbreads
Water
1 teaspoon olive oil
1 cup thinly sliced red onion
1 teaspoon salt
Pinch red pepper flakes
2 tablespoons honey
½ cup ricotta cheese
½ cup feta cheese
1 cup blueberries
1 cup baby arugula

Preparation
1. Preheat the oven to 400°F. Line a baking sheet with parchment paper.
2. Brush the flatbreads with water on both sides and place them on the prepared parchment paper.
3. In a medium skillet, heat the olive oil over medium-low heat. Add the onions and season with salt and red pepper flakes. Cook until they are translucent, about 5 minutes. Stir in the honey and remove the skillet from the heat.
4. Meanwhile, spread the ricotta and feta cheese over the bread. Top with the caramelized onions and blueberries. Bake for 10 minutes, or until the blueberries burst and the bread is toasted.
5. Remove from oven and enjoy the pizza warm with a generous sprinkle of arugula on top.

Nutritional Facts (355 g per single serving)
Calories 601
Fats 22 g
Carbs 84 g
Protein 23 g
Sodium 1984 mg

Mushroom and Blueberry Balsamic Pot Roast

Servings: 6

Ingredients
3 ½ pounds chuck roast
Salt and pepper, to taste
3 tablespoons olive oil, divided
2 white onions, quartered
6 carrots, peeled and cut into 2-inch slices
1 cup mushrooms, thickly sliced
4 cloves garlic, thinly sliced
½ cup balsamic vinegar
½ cup beef broth
¼ cup tomato sauce
2 cup fresh blueberries
3 sprigs fresh thyme
3 sprigs fresh rosemary

Preparation
1. Preheat the oven to 275°F. Season the roast with salt and pepper.
2. In a large Dutch oven or oven-safe pot, heat 1 tablespoon of oil over medium-high heat. Sear the meat for about a minute on each side, until browned. Transfer it to a clean plate.
3. Drizzle another tablespoon of oil into the pot. Add the onions and carrots and cook until brown on all sides, about 2-3 minutes. Transfer the vegetables to the same plate as the meat.

4. Add another tablespoon of oil. Cook the mushrooms and garlic until slightly browned, about 3 minutes. Remove them from the pot as well.
5. Pour in the balsamic vinegar, beef broth, tomato sauce, and blueberries. Using a wooden spoon, scrape the browned bits from the bottom of the pan, and bring the mixture to a boil. Reduce the heat to medium low and simmer for another 3-4 minutes, or until the berries are starting to burst. Using the back of the wooden spoon, mash the berries against the side of the pot to release their juices.
6. Return the cooked ingredients to the pot. Add the thyme and rosemary and cover with the lid.
7. Place the Dutch oven into the oven. Cook for about 3 hours, or until the meat is fork tender. Serve immediately on its own or with side dishes

Nutritional Facts (486 g per single serving)
Calories 540
Fats 24 g
Carbs 23 g
Protein 58 g
Sodium 364 mg

Flank Steak with Blueberry Sauce

Servings: 4

Ingredients
4 (6 ounce) flank steaks
Salt and pepper, to taste
2 tablespoons butter
2 tablespoons shallots, minced
2 cloves garlic, minced
1 cup beef stock
⅓ cup red wine
1 teaspoon fresh thyme, minced
1 cup fresh blueberries

Preparation
1. Season the steak with salt and pepper on both sides.
2. In a small saucepan, melt the butter over medium heat. Sauté the shallots and garlic until fragrant, about 1 minute.
3. Add the beef stock, wine, and thyme into the skillet. Reduce the heat to low and simmer for another 10 minutes. Taste and adjust the seasoning.
4. Heat a large skillet over medium-high heat. Sear the steaks for 3-4 minutes on each side, depending on the desired doneness. Remove the steaks to a clean serving platter.
5. Once all the steaks are cooked, pour the sauce into the steak skillet. Deglaze the pan by scraping the bottom with a wooden spoon. Add the blueberries and bring the sauce to a boil.

6. Serve the steak with a generous drizzle of the sauce.

Nutritional Facts (295 g per single serving)
Calories 379
Fats 20 g
Carbs 7 g
Protein 37 g
Sodium 218 mg

Juicy Blueberry Beef Burger

Servings: 4

Ingredients
2 slices whole wheat bread, crusts removed, torn into pieces
⅓ cup fresh blueberries
1 tablespoon balsamic vinegar
2 teaspoons Dijon mustard
1 teaspoon Worcestershire sauce
2 cloves garlic, minced
Pinch salt
Pepper, to taste
12 ounces 90% lean ground beef
Other ingredients: Burger patties, lettuce, tomato slices, cheese, and any desired toppings

Preparation
1. In a food processor, process the bread into fine crumbs, and transfer them to a large bowl.
2. In the same food processor, puree the blueberries, vinegar, mustard, Worcestershire sauce, garlic, salt, and pepper. Pour the sauce into the bowl with the breadcrumbs.
3. Add the ground beef to the bowl. Using a spatula, mix all the ingredients until they are thoroughly combined.
4. Divide the meat into 4 equal patties, ½-inch thick.
5. Preheat the grill to medium-high heat. Cook the patties until they are browned on the outside, about 3-4 minutes on each side. Serve immediately with buns and your favorite trimmings.

Nutritional Facts (123 g per single serving)
Calories 205
Fats 9 g
Carbs 10 g
Protein 19 g
Sodium 211 mg

Grilled Chicken with Blueberry Guacamole

Servings: 6

Ingredients
6 boneless skinless chicken breasts
1 ½ cups Greek yogurt
Juice of 2 limes
1 tablespoon cumin
1 teaspoon salt
2 cloves garlic
1 teaspoon chili powder
1 chipotle pepper
½ teaspoon adobo sauce

Guacamole:
5 avocados
1 cup blueberries
Juice of 2 limes
4 tablespoons cilantro, chopped
2 jalapeños, finely diced
Salt and pepper, to taste

Preparation
1. To make the marinade, blend the yogurt, lime juice, cumin, salt, garlic, chili powder, chipotle pepper, and adobo sauce in a food processor until it becomes smooth. Transfer the marinade to a plastic bag and add the chicken breasts. Give the bag a few good shakes to coat the chicken with the marinade. Place the bag in the refrigerator and allow to sit for at least 30 minutes.

2. Meanwhile, make the guacamole. Half the avocados and scoop the flesh out into a clean bowl. Stir in the blueberries, lime juice, cilantro, jalapeños, salt, and pepper. Mash all the ingredients with a fork. Refrigerate until ready to serve.
3. Preheat the grill to medium-high heat. Cook the meat for about 5-8 minutes per side, or until it is completely cooked through.
4. Serve the chicken with the blueberry guacamole on the side.

Nutritional Facts (572 g per single serving)
Calories 688
Fats 35 g
Carbs 24 g
Protein 71 g
Sodium 548 mg

Pork Chops with Tangy Blueberry Sauce

Servings: 4

Ingredients
4 boneless pork chops
Salt and pepper, to taste
2 tablespoons vegetable oil, divided
1 shallot, finely diced
½ cup red wine
¼ cup water
½ cup blueberries
Zest and juice of ½ a lemon
2 tablespoons unsalted butter
Fresh parsley, roughly chopped

Preparation
1. Preheat the oven to 425°F. Season the pork chops with salt and pepper on both sides.
2. In a large oven-proof skillet, heat 1 tablespoon of oil over medium-high heat. Once the oil starts shimmering, cook the pork chops for about 1 minute on each side, or until browned. Remove the skillet from the heat and continue cooking them in the oven for 10 minutes, until they are completely cooked through.
3. Meanwhile, make the sauce. In a small saucepan, heat the remaining oil over medium-high heat. Fry the shallot for about 2 minutes, until it becomes soft and brown. Pour in the wine and water and bring it to boil, about 2 minutes.

4. Pour the blueberries into the pan and simmer until they start bursting and releasing their juices. Add the zest and juice of half a lemon. Continue bubbling until the sauce starts to thicken to your desired consistency. Remove the pot from the heat and stir in the butter.
5. Once the pork chops are cooked, remove them from the oven. Allow the meat to rest for 5 minutes before serving.
6. Plate the meat with a heaping scoop of the tangy blueberry sauce, and a generous sprinkle of parsley.

Nutritional Facts *(267 g per single serving)*
Calories 436
Fats 26 g
Carbs 4 g
Protein 40 g
Sodium 92 mg

Broiled Salmon with Blueberry Glaze

Servings: 4

Ingredients
½ cup fresh blueberries
5 sprigs fresh thyme
1 tablespoon granulated sugar
1 tablespoon balsamic vinegar
2 teaspoons lemon juice
Salt and pepper, to taste
4 (4 ounce) salmon filets

Preparation
1. To make the glaze, combine the blueberries, thyme, sugar, balsamic vinegar, lemon juice and ¼ teaspoon of salt in a small saucepan. Bring the ingredients to boil over medium-high heat. Continue cooking until the blueberries start releasing their juices and the sauce thickens, about 15 minutes.
2. Preheat the broiler to high. Line a baking sheet with aluminum foil.
3. Arrange the salmon filets skin-side down on the baking sheet. Season with salt and pepper on both sides.
4. Generously brush the blueberry sauce on the salmon. Place it under the broiler for 3 minutes, then remove it from the oven and brush on another layer. Return it to the broiler for another 5 minutes, until it is completely cooked through.

Nutritional Facts (142 g per single serving)
Calories 188
Fats 8 g
Carbs 7 g
Protein 23 g
Sodium 51 mg

Appetizers and Snack Recipes
Blueberry Banana Muffins

Servings: 12

Ingredients
1 cup whole wheat flour
¾ cup all-purpose flour
¼ cup wheat germ
1 teaspoon baking soda
½ teaspoon salt
2 ripe bananas, mashed
⅓ cup 2% milk
1 teaspoon vanilla extract
1 stick unsalted butter, at room temperature
⅓ cup granulated sugar
⅓ cup packed light brown sugar
2 large eggs
1 cup frozen blueberries

Preparation
1. Preheat the oven to 350°F. Line a 12-cup muffin tin with paper liners.
2. In a medium bowl, whisk together the flour, wheat germ, baking soda, and salt.
3. In a separate bowl, mix the mashed bananas with milk and vanilla extract.
4. Using an electric hand mixer, beat the butter with the granulated and brown sugar until the mixture becomes light and fluffy. Add the eggs one at a time, making sure that the ingredients are fully incorporated with each addition.

5. Slowly mix in the flour and banana mixture, alternating between them. Beat until the ingredients are just combined with no visible lumps present in the batter. Using a spatula, fold in the blueberries.
6. Spoon the batter into the prepared muffin tin. Bake for 20-25 minutes, rotating once halfway through. To check for doneness, insert a skewer into the center of a muffin and it should come out clean.
7. Remove the muffin tin from the oven. Allow the muffins to cool in the tin for 10 minutes, before transferring them to a wire rack to cool down completely.

Nutritional Facts (70 g per single serving)
Calories 212
Fats 9 g
Carbs 28 g
Protein 4 g
Sodium 221 mg

Peach and Blueberry Salsa with Brie

Servings: 4

Ingredients
1 cup fresh blueberries
1 ripe peach, seeded and diced
½ jalapeño, diced
1 tablespoon mint, chopped
Juice of 1 lime
1 teaspoon fresh ginger, peeled and grated
1 tablespoon honey
Salt and pepper, to taste
1 small Brie wheel (about 5 inches)
Baguette, sliced, for serving

Preparation
1. Preheat the oven to 350°F. Line a baking sheet with parchment paper.
2. In a medium bowl, toss together the blueberries, peach, jalapeño, mint, lime juice, ginger, honey, salt, and pepper. Set the mixture aside for at least 15 minutes for the flavors to develop.
3. Place the Brie on the prepared baking tray, and bake for 5 minutes, or until the cheese is warm but still firm to touch
4. To serve, pile the warm Brie with the fruit salsa. Dip into the oozy cheese with the baguette slices.

Nutritional Facts (169 g per single serving)
Calories 315
Fats 9 g
Carbs 55 g
Protein 9 g
Sodium 203 mg

Blueberry Buttermilk Scones

Servings: 12

Ingredients
1 ½ cups all-purpose flour
½ cup cake flour
3 tablespoons granulated sugar
2 ½ teaspoons baking powder
¾ teaspoon salt
1 stick cold, unsalted butter, cubed
1 cup fresh blueberries
½ cup low-fat buttermilk
2 large eggs
½ teaspoon vanilla extract

Preparation
1. Preheat the oven to 375°F. Line a baking sheet with parchment paper.
2. In a food processor, mix the all-purpose flour, cake flour, sugar, baking powder, and salt. Add the cold butter cubes and give the ingredients a few pulses until the mixture reaches the texture of a coarse cornmeal. Tip it out into a large bowl.
3. Add the blueberries to the flour mixture and fold them in using a spatula.
4. In a separate bowl, whisk together the buttermilk, 1 egg, and the vanilla extract. Pour the wet ingredients into the dry ingredients and give it a gentle stir to just combine.
5. Transfer the dough to a work surface and roll it out to a 1-inch thick rectangle. Using a sharp knife, cut out 12 scone triangles. Transfer the scones to the prepared baking sheet.

6. In a small bowl, crack the remaining egg and beat it lightly. Brush the top of the scones with the egg wash.
7. Bake the scones for 20 minutes, or until the tops are golden brown. Transfer them to a wire rack to cool completely.

Nutritional Facts (65 g per single serving)
Calories 173
Fats 9 g
Carbs 20 g
Protein 4 g
Sodium 181 mg

Blueberry and Lemon Squares

Servings: 18 squares

Ingredients
1 ¼ cups walnuts
¼ cup sunflower seeds
1 ½ cups dates
½ cup dried blueberries
1 teaspoon lemon zest

Preparation
1. Line a 9x5 loaf pan with parchment paper.
2. In a food processor, blend all the ingredients until a paste forms.
3. Transfer the mixture to the prepared loaf pan. Press the mixture evenly into the pan.
4. Refrigerate the pan for a day.
5. Remove the bars from the pan and discard the parchment paper. Cut the bar into 18 squares. Store the squares in a container in the fridge.

Nutritional Facts (27 g per single serving)
Calories 115
Fats 7 g
Carbs 14 g
Protein 2 g
Sodium 1 mg

Yogurt-Coated Blueberry Bites

Servings: 12

Ingredients
1 pint container blueberries
1 cup vanilla, non-fat Greek yogurt
1 tablespoon honey

Preparation
1. Line a baking sheet with parchment paper.
2. In a mixing bowl, combine the yogurt and honey together.
3. Add the blueberries to the yogurt mixture, and gently stir the blueberries to coat each one with the yogurt. Using a fork, scoop each blueberry out and tap the excess yogurt away.
4. Arrange each blueberry on the prepared parchment paper, making sure they do not touch each other. Place the baking sheet into the freezer for about an hour, or until the blueberries are frozen.
5. Enjoy them cold, and store the leftovers in an airtight container in the freezer.

Nutritional Facts (27 g per single serving)
Calories 39
Fats 0 g
Carbs 9 g
Protein 2 g
Sodium 8 mg

Blueberry Frozen Yogurt Ice Cream

Makes: 1 quart

Ingredients
2 cups full-fat Greek yogurt
2 ½ cups fresh blueberries
⅔ cup honey
Juice and zest of 1 lemon

Preparation
1. In a medium saucepan, combine the blueberries, honey, and lemon zest and juice. Heat the mixture up to a simmer over medium heat, and cook for 15 minutes. During the cooking, use the back of a wooden spoon to press the berries against the side of the pot to help them release their juices. Once the mixture thickens to a syrupy consistency, remove the pot from the heat and allow it to cool completely.
2. For a smoother ice cream, strain the mixture through a fine mesh sieve to remove the skin and solid pieces. Use a spoon or fork to press as much liquid through the sieve as possible.
3. Once the blueberry mixture is cooled to room temperature, place it in the refrigerator to chill at least 4 hours, or overnight.
1. Spoon the yogurt and blueberry mixture into your ice cream maker and prepare it according to the manufacturer's instructions. Serve immediately, or transfer it to a container to freeze for a few hours.

Nutritional Facts (1214 g per single serving)
Calories 1464
Fats 21 g
Carbs 267 g
Protein 55 g
Sodium 214 mg

Almond Blueberry Oat Bites

Servings: 12

Ingredients
2 cups rolled oats
2 tablespoons flaxseed meal
⅓ cup sliced almonds
2 tablespoons peanut butter
1 tablespoon vanilla extract
2 tablespoons honey
¼ teaspoon cinnamon
½ teaspoon salt
1 teaspoon baking powder
1 egg
¾ cup almond milk
½ cup fresh blueberries
Non-stick cooking spray

Preparation
1. Preheat the oven to 350°F. Grease a 12-cup muffin pan with non-stick cooking spray.
2. In a large bowl, mix together the oats, flaxseed meal, almonds, peanut butter, vanilla extract, honey, cinnamon, salt, and baking powder.
3. In a separate bowl, whisk the egg with the almond milk. Combine the egg mixture with the oat mixture and stir to make sure it is well incorporated. Fold in the blueberries.
4. Divide the batter evenly into each of the muffin holes, filling each one about ¾ full.

5. Bake for 20 minutes, or until they are golden brown. Remove them from the oven and let them cool in the pan for 5 minutes, then transfer them to a wire rack to cool completely. Serve immediately, or keep them for up to 5 days in the refrigerator.

Nutritional Facts (65 g per single serving)
Calories 146
Fats 4 g
Carbs 22 g
Protein 6 g
Sodium 116 mg

Blueberry Sunflower Energy Balls

Servings: 14 bites

Ingredients
¼ cup raw cashews
6 Medjool dates, pitted
¾ cup dried blueberries
⅓ cup sunflower seed butter, or any other nut or seed butter
½ teaspoon spirulina powder
½ teaspoon cinnamon
Pinch sea salt
Optional: Sesame seeds, to coat

Preparation
1. In a food processor, give the cashews a few quick pulses until they are the consistency of a fine crumb.
2. Add the dates, blueberries, sunflower seed butter, spirulina powder, cinnamon, and salt. Blend until the mixture forms a paste.
3. Divide the paste into 14 equal portions and roll them into balls. Coat the outside with sesame seeds, if desired.
4. Enjoy immediately or keep refrigerated until ready to consume.

Nutritional Facts (29 g per single serving)
Calories 114
Fats 12 g
Carbs 11 g
Protein 2 g
Sodium 12 mg

Chewy Blueberry Gummies

Servings: 9

Ingredients
⅔ cup lemon juice
1 cup fresh blueberries
4 tablespoons unflavored gelatin

Preparation
1. In a medium saucepan, heat the lemon juice and blueberries over medium heat. Cook until the lemon juice starts to steam.
2. Pour the heated mixture into a blender or food processor. Mix until it becomes smooth.
3. Add the gelatin to the mixture and give it another pulse.
4. Transfer the mixture to a 9x9 glass dish. Place it in the refrigerator for at least 30 minutes to let the gelatin set.
5. Cut into 9 equal squares.

Nutritional Facts (38 g per single serving)
Calories 24
Fats 0 g
Carbs 4 g
Protein 3 g
Sodium 7 mg

Blueberry Coconut Bars

Servings: 16

Ingredients
4 cups rolled oats
¼ cup whole wheat flour
½ cup shredded coconut
⅓ cup light brown sugar
½ teaspoon salt
1 cup dried blueberries
½ cup coconut oil, melted
½ cup honey
1 ½ teaspoons coconut extract
½ teaspoon vanilla extract

Preparation
1. Preheat the oven to 350°F. Line a 9x13 baking pan with parchment paper.
2. In a large bowl, mix the oats, flour, shredded coconut, sugar, salt, and blueberries.
3. In a separate bowl, whisk the oil, honey, coconut extract, and vanilla extract together. Add the wet ingredients to the dry ingredients, and mix thoroughly to combine.
4. Transfer the mixture to the prepared pan and press it down firmly. Bake for 40 minutes, or until the top is golden brown. Remove it from oven and allow to cool completely.
5. Cut into 16 equal bars, and serve.

Nutritional Facts (79 g per single serving)
Calories 330
Fats 15 g
Carbs 49 g
Protein 8 g
Sodium 78 mg

Dessert Recipes
Baked Cheesecake with Blueberry Compote

Servings: 12

Ingredients
1 ½ cups graham cracker crumbs
¾ stick unsalted butter, melted
1 ½ cups + 3 tablespoons granulated sugar, divided
2 ½ pounds cream cheese, at room temperature (5 8-ounce packages)
¼ cup sour cream
7 large eggs
1 ½ teaspoons vanilla extract
4 cups frozen blueberries
2 teaspoons cornstarch
¼ cup water
1 tablespoon lemon juice

Preparation
1. Preheat the oven to 350°F. Lightly grease the bottom of a 9-inch spring form pan.
2. In a small bowl, mix together the graham cracker crumbs, melted butter and 1 tablespoon of sugar. Press the mixture down into the bottom of the pan using the back of a spoon. Bake for 8 minutes, and let it cool down completely
3. Increase the oven temperature to 450°F. Adjust the oven rack to the lower third of the oven.
4. In the bowl of an electric stand mixer, beat the cream cheese and 1 ½ cups of sugar on medium-high speed until it is light and fluffy, about 2-3

minutes. Using a spatula, scrape down the sides of the bowl to make sure all the cream is incorporated.
5. Reduce the mixer's speed to medium. Combine the eggs one at a time into the filling, making sure the ingredients are well incorporated with each addition.
6. Lower the mixer's speed to low. Add the sour cream and vanilla extract, and mix until there are no visible streaks. Transfer the batter to the pie crust.
7. Bake the pie at 450°F for 15 minutes. After that, reduce the oven temperature to 225°F, and continue baking for about 1 ¼ hours, or until the center is set. While baking, avoid opening the oven to prevent the cake from cracking.
8. Once the cake is done baking, turn off the oven but do not remove the cheesecake. Leave the oven door ajar for 15 minutes. After 15 minutes, remove the cake from the oven and leave it to cool at room temperature, then place it in the refrigerator to let it chill and set completely.
9. Meanwhile, make the blueberry compote. Combine the cornstarch, lemon juice, water and 2 tablespoons of sugar in a medium saucepan. Heat the mixture over medium heat until the liquid starts to thicken. Stir in the blueberries and cook until bubbles start to form. Remove the pot from the heat and set it aside to cool down completely.
10. When ready to serve, run an offset spatula or butter knife around the side of the pan to help release the cake.
11. Serve the cake with a scoop of blueberry sauce on it.

Nutritional Facts (233 g per single serving)
Calories 616
Fats 44 g
Carbs 49 g
Protein 11 g
Sodium 372 mg

Classic Blueberry Pie

Servings: 10

Ingredients
Pie crust:
2 ½ cups all-purpose flour
1 teaspoon salt
1 tablespoon sugar
1 cup cold unsalted butter, cubed
½-⅓ cup ice cold water

Filling:
12 ounces fresh blueberries
½ cup + 1 tablespoon granulated sugar
¼ cup cornstarch
1 tablespoon lemon juice
1 tablespoon cold unsalted butter, cubed
1 large egg yolk
1 tablespoon heavy cream
Demerara sugar

Preparation
1. In a food processor, pulse together the flour, salt, and sugar. Throw in the cold butter cubes and process until it reaches the consistency of wet sand. With the blades still moving, drizzle in the cold water so all the ingredients can come together to form a dough.
2. Divide the dough into two equal portions, each flattened to form a 6-inch disc. Wrap the discs with plastic film, and refrigerate them for 15 minutes.

3. Meanwhile, prepare the pie filling. Toss together the blueberries, sugar, cornstarch, and lemon juice in a large bowl. Using your fingers or a fork, gently crush some of the blueberries. Set the mixture aside and allow it to soften for 15 minutes.
4. To make the pie shell, lightly flour a piece of parchment paper and roll out one of the discs to about 11 inches wide. Flip the dough onto a 9-inch pie dish, and press it into the bottom and sides of the plate. Trim off the excess dough, leaving behind about ½ an inch hanging from the lip of the pie dish.
5. Roll out the second piece of dough to about as big as the previous pie shell. Using a sharp knife, cut it into 1-inch thick strips.
6. To assemble, fill the pie shell with the blueberry filling, and shape it into a mound. Place the cold butter cubes in the center of the mound.
7. To make the lattice top, lay 5 pie strips on top of the filling, making sure they are equally spaced. Take a new dough strip and place it perpendicular to original 5 strips. Take the 2nd and 4th strips and arrange them under the new dough strip. Next, take a new dough strip and repeat the same steps, except this time, place the 1st, 3rd and 5th strips under the new dough strip. Cover the top with this lattice pattern, and trim off all excess dough. Tuck the dough strips under the pie shell, and crimp the edges with your fingers.
8. In a small bowl, whisk together the egg yolk and cream to create an egg wash. Brush the top and edges of the pie with the egg wash and sprinkle some demerara sugar over it. Keep the pie in the fridge for 30 minutes for the pie to firm up.

9. Preheat the oven to 425°F. Place the rack in the bottom third of the oven.
10. Cover the pie with foil, and bake for 20 minutes. Lower the oven temperature to 350°F, remove the foil, and cover the pie with a piece of parchment paper. Halfway through baking, rotate the pie dish. Bake until the dough turns golden brown and the blueberry filling becomes thick and bubbly, about 60-70 minutes. Remove the pie from the oven, and allow it to cool for 3-4 hours before serving.

Nutritional Facts (110 g per single serving)
Calories 371
Fats 21 g
Carbs 43 g
Protein 4 g
Sodium 238 mg

Blueberry Bread Pudding

Servings: 6

Ingredients
1 (16 ounce) loaf French bread, cubed
8 ounces cream cheese, cut into pieces
3 cups fresh blueberries, divided
6 large eggs
4 cups milk
½ cup sugar
¼ cup butter, melted
¼ cup maple syrup
10 ounces blueberry preserves

Preparation
1. The night before, line the bottom of a 9x13 baking dish with half the bread cubes. Scatter the cream cheese pieces and 1 cup of the blueberries over, and then top it with the remaining bread cubes.
2. Whisk the eggs, milk, sugar, butter, and maple syrup in a medium bowl.
3. Pour the wet ingredients into the bread mixture, and give it a good toss. Cover with aluminum foil and refrigerate it overnight.
4. When you are ready to cook, preheat the oven to 350°F. Bake the bread pudding with the foil for 30 minutes. Remove the foil and continue baking for another 30 minutes, or until the top is lightly browned.
5. While the bread pudding is cooking, combine 2 cups of fresh blueberries and the blueberry preserves in a small saucepan. Heat it over low heat until it becomes warm and bubbly.

6. Serve the bread pudding warm with a generous drizzle of blueberry sauce over it.

Nutritional Facts (332 g per single serving)
Calories 669
Fats 19 g
Carbs 81 g
Protein 18 g
Sodium 469 mg

Blueberry Coffee Cake

Servings: 8

Ingredients
1 cup butter, softened
2 cups granulated sugar
2 large eggs
1 cup sour cream
1 teaspoon vanilla extract
1 ⅝ cups all-purpose flour
1 teaspoon baking powder
¼ teaspoon salt
1 cup fresh or frozen blueberries
½ cup brown sugar
1 teaspoon ground cinnamon
½ cup pecans, chopped
Non-stick cooking spray

Preparation
1. Preheat the oven to 350°F. Grease a 9-inch Bundt pan with non-stick cooking spray and lightly dust it with flour.
2. In the bowl of an electric stand mixer, beat the butter and sugar on medium-high speed until it becomes light and fluffy, about 2-3 minutes. Add the eggs one at a time, making sure the first is fully incorporated before adding the next. Reduce the speed to medium and mix in the sour cream and vanilla extract.
3. Turn the speed to low. Add the flour, baking powder, and salt and combine until a smooth batter is formed. Using a spatula, fold in the blueberries.

4. In a small bowl, whisk together the brown sugar, cinnamon, and pecans.
5. Pour half the batter into the prepared pan, and scatter half the sugar mixture over the batter. Cover with the rest of the batter and the rest of the sugar mixture. Swirl the layers together with a butter knife.
6. Bake for about an hour, or until a skewer inserted in the thickest part of the cake comes out clean.
7. Remove the cake from the oven and let it cool completely on a wire rack. To serve, place a plate over the top of the Bundt pan and flip it over.

Nutritional Facts (180 g per single serving)
Calories 657
Fats 35 g
Carbs 84 g
Protein 6 g
Sodium 107 mg

Blueberry and Buttermilk Tart

Servings: 12

Ingredients
1 cup all-purpose flour
¼ cup + ⅓ cup sugar
½ teaspoon coarse salt
½ cup cold unsalted butter, cubed
⅓ cup whole almonds
1 teaspoon unflavored gelatin
1 tablespoon cold water
½ cup heavy cream
3 tablespoons sugar
⅛ teaspoon salt
1 cup low-fat buttermilk
1 tablespoon fresh lemon juice
3 cups fresh blueberries

Preparation
1. In a food processor, pulse together the flour, ¼ cup of sugar, and coarse salt. With the motor still running, add the cold butter cubes and mix until it reaches a wet sand consistency. Gently press it together, and shape it into a disc.
2. To the food processor, add ⅓ cup of sugar and the almonds. Blend until they are finely ground.
3. Sprinkle half the almond sugar mixture on a work surface. Place the dough on top of the mixture, and roll it out to an 11-inch square. Scatter the remaining almond sugar mixture on top of the dough.

4. Transfer the dough to a 9x9 tart pan. Press the dough to the bottom and sides of the pan, and trim off any excess. Refrigerate the tart shell for at least 30 minutes.
5. Meanwhile, preheat the oven to 325°F. Bake the tart shell for about 30 minutes, or until it is golden brown. Remove it from the oven and let it cool completely.
6. To make the filling, start by preparing the gelatin mix. In a small bowl, combine the gelatin with the cold water. Let it sit for at least 5 minutes.
7. Meanwhile, combine the cream, 3 tablespoons of sugar, and salt in a small saucepan. Heat the mixture over medium heat to dissolve the sugar. Pour the gelatin mixture into the warm cream and give it a good stir, until it is fully incorporated. Remove the pot from the heat and pour in the buttermilk and lemon juice.
8. Gently release the tart from the pan. Transfer the custard to the tart and spread it out. Refrigerate for about 15 minutes before topping it with the rest of the blueberries. Return it to the fridge and chill for another 2 hours for it to firm up.

Nutritional Facts (105 g per single serving)
Calories 233
Fats 14 g
Carbs 29 g
Protein 3 g
Sodium 141 mg

Blueberry Ice Pops

Servings: 8

Ingredients
3 cups fresh or frozen blueberries
¾ cup sugar
½ cup water
⅓ cup fresh lime juice

Preparation
1. In a large saucepan, heat the blueberries, sugar, and water over medium heat, until the berries have burst, about 5 minutes. Remove the pot from the heat and set it aside to cool down.
2. Spoon the berry mixture and lime juice into a blender, and puree until it is smooth.
3. Pour the mixture into molds and insert wooden sticks. Freeze the ice pops for at least 3 hours.

Nutritional Facts (99 g per single serving)
Calories 107
Fats 0 g
Carbs 28 g
Protein 0 g
Sodium 1 mg

Blueberry Swirl Cupcakes

Servings: 12

Ingredients
1 ⅔ cups cake flour
¼ teaspoon baking soda
1 teaspoon baking powder
½ teaspoon salt
1 stick unsalted butter, at room temperature
6 tablespoons + ⅔ cup granulated sugar
2 large eggs
1 teaspoon vanilla extract
¾ cup sour cream
1 ¼ cups blueberries
¼ cup dark-brown sugar
1 teaspoon cinnamon

Icing:
1 ¼ sticks unsalted butter, softened
8 ounces cream cheese, at room temperature
½ teaspoon vanilla extract
2 ⅔ cups confectioners' sugar, sifted
¼ cup blueberry jam

Preparation
1. Preheat the oven to 375°F. Line a 12-hole muffin tin with cupcake liners.
2. Whisk together the flour, baking soda, baking powder, and salt.
3. Using an electric hand mixer, cream the butter and ⅔ cup sugar together on medium-high speed until it becomes light and fluffy, 2-3 minutes.

4. Add the eggs one at a time, making sure all the ingredients are well incorporated with each addition. Pour in the vanilla extract, and scrape down the sides if necessary.
5. Reduce the speed to low. Add ⅓ of the flour mixture, followed by ¼ cup of sour cream, and continue alternating between them until all the ingredients are used up. Using a spatula, fold in the blueberries.
6. Portion an equal amount of batter for the cupcakes, filling each to about ¾ full.
7. Whisk the 6 tablespoons of granulated sugar, brown sugar, and cinnamon in a small bowl. Scatter the sugar mixture on top of each cupcake.
8. Bake the cupcakes for about 20 minutes, or until they are golden brown and a toothpick inserted in the center comes out clean. Remove the cupcakes from the oven and allow them to cool on a wire rack.
9. To make the icing, cream together the butter and cream cheese using an electric hand mixer set to medium-high speed. Beat until it turns light and fluffy, about 2-3 minutes.
10. Reduce the speed to low, and slowly incorporate the confectioners' sugar and vanilla extract. Once all the ingredients are mixed in, increase the speed to medium-high and beat for another minute to lighten the mixture. Add the blueberry jam to the icing and stir it in.
11. Transfer the icing to a piping bag with the tip snipped off. Pipe the icing on top of each cupcake. Enjoy immediately, or store in the fridge for up to a day.

Nutritional Facts (144 g per single serving)
Calories 507
Fats 28 g
Carbs 63 g
Protein 4 g
Sodium 283 mg

Blueberry Cobbler

Servings: 8

Ingredients
1 ¼ cups all-purpose flour
½ cup + ⅓ cup sugar
¼ teaspoon salt
1 ½ teaspoons baking powder
¾ cup milk
⅓ cup butter, melted
2 cups fresh blueberries
Non-stick cooking spray
Topping: vanilla or blueberry ice cream

Preparation
1. Preheat the oven to 350°F. Lightly grease an 8-inch square pan with non-stick cooking spray.
2. Whisk together the flour, ½ cup of sugar, salt, and baking powder.
3. Pour the milk and butter into the dry ingredients, and stir to combine.
4. Transfer the mixture to the prepared pan. Scatter the blueberries and ⅓ cup of sugar all over the mixture. Bake for 40-45 minutes, or until a toothpick inserted into the dough comes out clean.
5. Remove the pan from the oven and allow it to rest for 5 minutes. The cobbler is best served warm on its own, or with a scoop of ice-cream.

Nutritional Facts (119 g per single serving)
Calories 288
Fats 9 g
Carbs 51 g
Protein 3 g
Sodium 85 mg

Lemon Blueberry Pound Cake

Servings: 8

Ingredients
2 ½ cups flour
2 teaspoons baking powder
1 teaspoon salt
1 cup butter, at room temperature
1 ¾ cups sugar
Zest of one lemon
3 large eggs
½ teaspoon vanilla extract
¾ cup buttermilk
3 cups fresh blueberries
Non-stick cooking spray

Glaze:
1 ½ cups powdered sugar
1 tablespoon lemon juice
1 tablespoon lemon zest
1 tablespoon milk
¼ teaspoon vanilla

Preparation
1. Preheat the oven to 350°F. Lightly grease two loaf pans with non-stick cooking spray.
2. Whisk together the flour, baking powder, and salt.
3. In a separate bowl, beat the butter, sugar, and lemon zest with an electric hand mixer until they become light and fluffy, 2-3 minutes. Add the eggs one at a time, making sure all the ingredients are incorporated with each addition. Stir in the vanilla.

4. Add the dry ingredients and buttermilk to the batter in batches, alternating between them. Fold in the blueberries using a spatula.
5. Transfer the batter to the prepared pans. Bake for an hour, rotating once halfway through. Remove the cakes from the oven and let them cool in the pans for 15 minutes. Run a knife around the edges to release the cakes, and allow them to cool completely on a wire rack.
6. Meanwhile, make the glaze. In a small bowl, whisk together all the ingredients until smooth. Drizzle the glaze all over the cooled pound cakes.

Nutritional Facts (211 g per single serving)
Calories 590
Fats 26 g
Carbs 84 g
Protein 8 g
Sodium 348 mg

Blackberry and Blueberry Turnovers

Servings: 6

Ingredients
¾ cup fresh or frozen blueberries
¾ cup fresh or frozen blackberries, halved
3 tablespoons sugar
2 teaspoons ginger, peeled and finely grated
2 teaspoons fresh lime juice
¼ teaspoon salt
2 tablespoons all-purpose flour
1 large egg, lightly beaten
¼ cup heavy cream
1 store-bought pie dough

Preparation
1. Preheat the oven to 350°F. Line a baking tray with parchment paper.
2. In a medium bowl, mix the blueberries, blackberries, sugar, ginger, lime juice, salt, and flour together.
3. In a small bowl, whisk the egg and heavy cream until smooth.
4. Roll out the pie dough to form a 15x10-inch rectangle. Cut the dough lengthwise into two halves, and further cut each half into 3 squares. You should get six equal squares in the end.
5. Scoop ¼ cup of the berry filling into each square. Brush the edges of each with the egg mixture. Fold one corner of the square to the opposite corner to form a triangle. Using a fork, crimp the edges to seal the turnover, and transfer it to the prepared baking tray.

6. Brush the top of the pastries with the egg wash, and poke a hole to allow steam to be released. Repeat until all 6 turnovers are made.
7. Bake for 35-45 minutes, or until the pastries are golden brown. Transfer them to a wire rack to cool slightly before enjoying them warm.

Nutritional Facts (96 g per single serving)
Calories 232
Fats 12 g
Carbs 28 g
Protein 4 g
Sodium 230 mg

Drink Recipes

Blueberry Ice Lemon Tea

Servings: 6-8

Ingredients
1 pound frozen blueberries
½ cup fresh lemon juice
4 cups water
10 tea bags, green or chamomile
¾ cup sugar
Garnish: Fresh blueberries

Preparation
1. In a large saucepan, bring the blueberries and lemon juice to a boil over medium heat. Lower the heat to low and continue simmering for about 10 minutes. During the cooking, use a wooden spoon to mash the berries slightly, to help them release their juices. Remove the pot from the heat and run the mixture through a fine mesh sieve to remove any solid pieces. Set it aside to cool down.
2. In another saucepan, bring the water to a boil over high heat. Add the tea bags and lower the heat to medium. Let the tea bags steep for 5-10 minutes, depending on the desired intensity of tea flavor. Remove the tea bags and pour the tea into a jug.
3. Stir in the sugar and blueberry mixture, and mix until all the sugar is dissolved. Cover the jug and allow it to rest for an hour. Serve with ice and fresh blueberries for garnish.

Nutritional Facts (252 g per single serving based on 6 cups)
Calories 127
Fats 0 g
Carbs 32 g
Protein 0 g
Sodium 1 mg

Chocolate Blueberry Smoothie

Servings: 2

Ingredients
1 cup frozen blueberries
2 teaspoons cocoa powder
1 cup almond milk, or any desired milk
¼ teaspoon vanilla extract
2 teaspoons maple syrup

Preparation
1. In a blender, mix all the ingredients until smooth.
2. Serve immediately, or pour the drink through a fine mesh sieve to remove any solids.
3. Serve cold.

Nutritional Facts (213 g per single serving)
Calories 84
Fats 2 g
Carbs 18 g
Protein 2 g
Sodium 96 mg

Blueberry Pineapple Mojito

Servings: 1

Ingredients
½ cup crushed ice
1 lime wedge
4-5 fresh mint leaves
2 tablespoons fresh blueberries
2-3 fresh pineapple chunks
1 tablespoon sugar
1 shot (1 ½ ounces) white rum
8 ounces soda water

Preparation
1. Put the lime wedge and sugar in a cocktail shaker. Muddle the ingredients to release the lime juice.
2. Rub the mint leaves between your fingers to release the aroma. Add the bruised mint, blueberries, and pineapple to the shaker. Use the muddler to push them into the lime juice.
3. Add the crushed ice and rum. Give it a good shake until all the sugar is dissolved.
4. Pour the contents into a glass and finish the drink off with soda water.

Nutritional Facts (384 g per single serving)
Calories 159
Fats 0 g
Carbs 16 g
Protein 0 g
Sodium 50 mg

Blueberry Ginger Bellini

Servings: 4

Ingredients
½ cup fresh blueberries
1 tablespoon minced ginger
1 tablespoon sugar
Juice of ½ a lemon
2 cups blueberry juice
2 cups sparkling wine

Preparation
1. Place the blueberries, ginger, sugar, and lemon juice in a cocktail shaker. Use a muddler to gently bruise them to release their juices.
2. Pour the blueberry juice into the shaker and allow it to steep for 5 minutes.
3. Strain away the solids and transfer the mixture to 4 champagne flutes.
4. Top up each glass with sparkling wine.

Nutritional Facts (253 g per single serving)
Calories 164
Fats 0 g
Carbs 27 g
Protein 1 g
Sodium 3 mg

Red Wine Blueberry and Peach Sangria

Servings: 4

Ingredients
½ cup water
½ cup white sugar
1 cup fresh blueberries
1 bottle dry red wine
⅓ cup Triple Sec
¼ cup brandy
1 orange, thinly sliced with peel on
1 peach, pitted and thinly sliced

Preparation
1. In a small saucepan, heat the water and sugar over medium heat. Stir occasionally until all the sugar is dissolved. Remove it from the heat and allow it to cool completely.
2. In a pitcher, mix the sugar syrup and blueberries. Using a large wooden spoon, gently muddle the blueberries to help release their juices.
3. Pour the wine, Triple Sec, brandy, and fruit slices into the pitcher. Cover and refrigerate for 4 hours, or overnight, to infuse the flavors.

Nutritional Facts (401 g per single serving)
Calories 407
Fats 0 g
Carbs 53 g
Protein 1 g
Sodium 9 mg

Condiment, Dressing, and Sauce Recipes

Blueberry Chia Seed Jam

Servings: 1 cup

Ingredients
3 cups fresh blueberries
3 tablespoons maple syrup
2 tablespoons chia seeds
½ teaspoon vanilla extract

Preparation
1. In a medium non-stick saucepan, mix the blueberries and maple syrup. Bring the mixture to a gentle boil on medium heat. Reduce the heat to medium low, and simmer for another 5 minutes. While cooking, use a wooden spoon to gently press the blueberries against the sides of the pot to help release their juices.
2. Spoon the chia seeds into the jam and stir it frequently. Cook until the jam thickens and reaches the desired consistency. Remove it from the heat.
3. Add the vanilla extract and allow the jam to cool down completely, as it continues to thicken during the process. Store the jam in the refrigerator for up to a week.

Nutritional Facts (539 g per single serving)
Calories 583
Fats 25 g
Carbs 131 g
Protein 9 g
Sodium 19 mg

Blueberry Chipotle Chutney

Servings: 4 cups

Ingredients
4 cups fresh blueberries
1 cup finely chopped Granny Smith apple
½ cup white wine vinegar
⅓ cup sugar
⅓ cup honey
3 tablespoons grated orange zest
1 tablespoon mustard seeds
2 tablespoons chopped canned chipotle chilies in adobo sauce (about 2 chilies)
½ teaspoon salt

Preparation
1. Combine all the ingredients in a large saucepan. Bring it to a boil over medium-high heat. Reduce the heat to medium low, and simmer, uncovered, for 25 minutes or until the mixture has a thick consistency.
2. Remove it from the heat and allow it to cool down. Store the chutney in an airtight container in the refrigerator for up to 2 months.

Nutritional Facts (271 g per single serving)
Calories 310
Fats 1 g
Carbs 79 g
Protein 2 g
Sodium 295 mg

Blueberry Cheddar Dip

Servings: 4

Ingredients
8 ounces cream cheese, softened
8 ounces white cheddar cheese, freshly grated
¼ teaspoon nutmeg
1 cup fresh blueberries

Preparation
1. Preheat the oven to 350°F.
2. In a bowl, mix together both cheeses, nutmeg, and blueberries. Transfer the mixture to an oven-safe bowl, and bake for 30-35 minutes, until the cheese becomes hot and bubbly.

Nutritional Facts (151 g per single serving)
Calories 449
Fats 39 g
Carbs 11 g
Protein 17 g
Sodium 549 mg

Blueberry Dessert Sauce

Servings: 1 cup

Ingredients
2 tablespoons unsalted butter, at room temperature
¼ cup white sugar
1 pint fresh blueberries

Preparation
1. In a small saucepan, melt the butter over medium heat.
2. Add the blueberries and sugar. Cook the mixture until the blueberries release their juices and become syrupy, about 2 minutes. Best served warm.

Nutritional Facts (326 g per single serving)
Calories 451
Fats 19 g
Carbs 76 g
Protein 2 g
Sodium 7 mg

Blueberry Vinaigrette

Servings: 4

Ingredients
4 tablespoons white wine vinegar
4 tablespoons warm vegetable broth
2-3 tablespoons water
1 teaspoon sugar
2 tablespoons olive oil
1 shallot, peeled and finely diced
⅓ cup fresh blueberries
Salt and pepper, to taste

Preparation
1. In a bowl, whisk together the vinegar, vegetable broth, water, and sugar. Slowly drizzle in the olive oil while continuously stirring the vinaigrette.
2. Stir in the shallot and blueberries. Season with salt and pepper to taste.

Nutritional Facts (68 g per single serving)
Calories 134
Fats 13 g
Carbs 5 g
Protein 0 g
Sodium 51 mg

Conclusion

As we have seen, blueberries are a valuable addition to our diet. They are rich in cancer-killing and heart-healing micronutrients, and delicious as well! We hope this collection of recipes will help you find ways to include them in your regular rotation of recipes, and your repertoire of special dishes! We know your family and friends will love them.

About the Author

Sarah Spencer, who lives in Canada with her husband and two children, describes herself as an avid foodie who prefers watching the Food Network over a hockey game or NCIS! She is a passionate cook who dedicates all her time between creating new recipes, writing cookbooks, and her family, though not necessarily in that order!

Sarah has had two major influences in her life regarding cooking, her Grandmother and Mama Li.

She was introduced to cooking at an early age by her Grandmother who thought cooking for your loved ones was the single most important thing in life. Not only that, but she was the World's Best Cook in the eyes of all those lucky enough to taste her well-kept secret recipes. Over the years, she conveyed her knowledge and appreciation of food to Sarah.

Sarah moved to Philadelphia when her father was transferred there when Sarah was a young teenager. She became close friends with a girl named Jade, whose parents owned a Chinese take-out restaurant. This is when Sarah met her second biggest influence, Mama Li. Mama Li was Jade's mother and a professional cook in her own restaurant. Sarah would spend many hours in the restaurant as a helper to Mama Li. Her first job was in the restaurant. Mama Li showed Sarah all about cooking Asian food, knife handling, and mixing just the right amount of spices. Sarah became an excellent Asian cook, especially in Chinese and Thai food.

Along the way, Sarah developed her own style in the kitchen. She loves to try new flavors and mix up ingredients in new and innovative ways. She is also very sensitive to her son's allergy to gluten and has been cooking gluten-free and paleo recipes for quite some time.

More Books from Sarah Spencer

Shown below are some of her other books. To check any of them out, just click on the book cover you like. Follow Sarah and join in her great love of cooking!

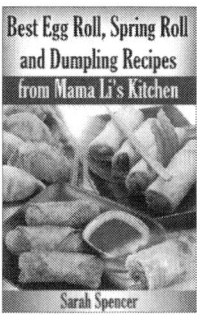 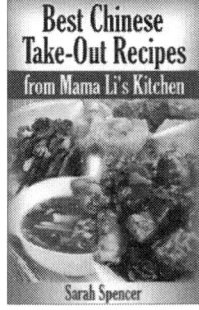 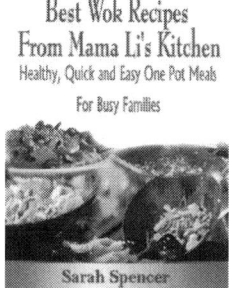

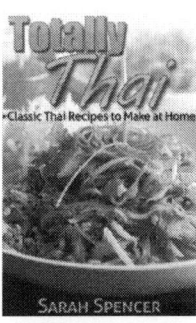 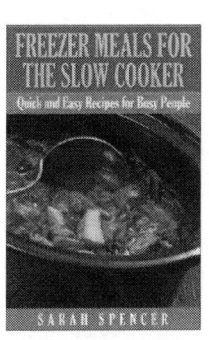 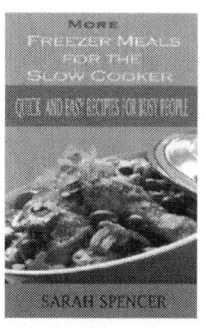

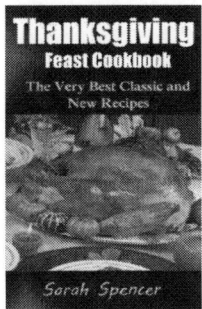 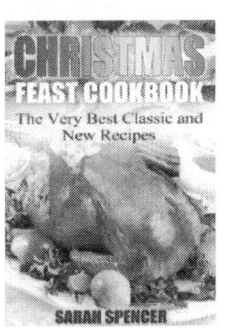 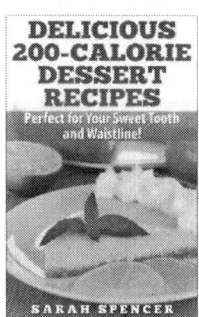

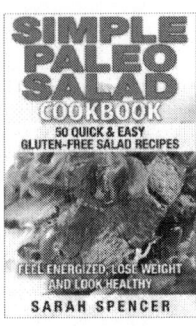
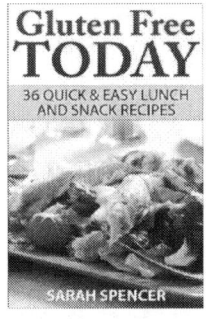
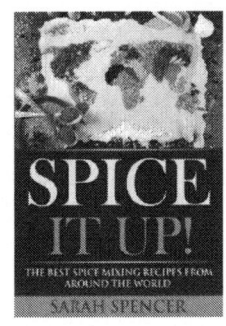
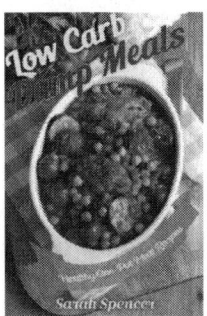
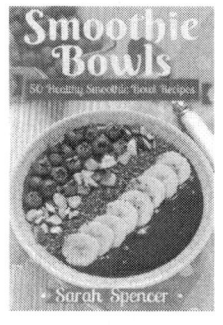
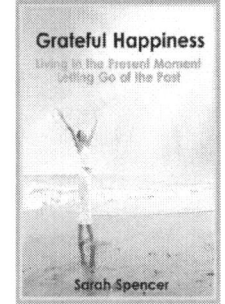
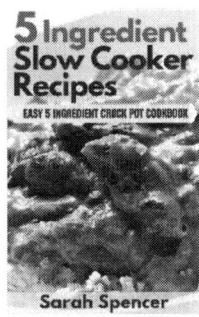
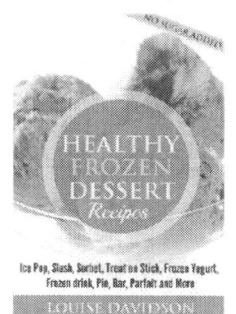
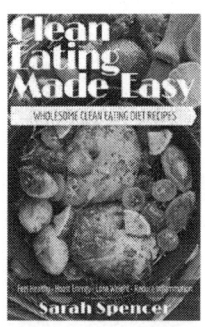
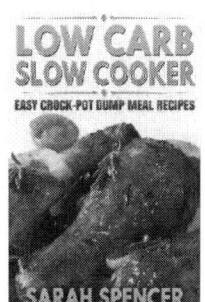
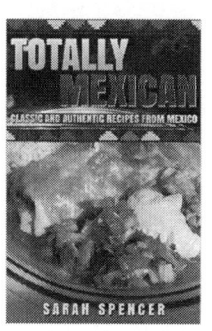
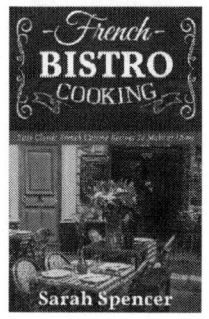

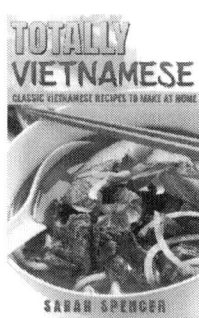
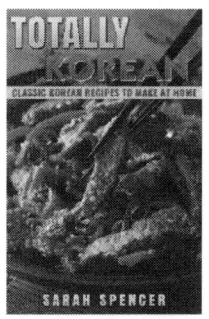
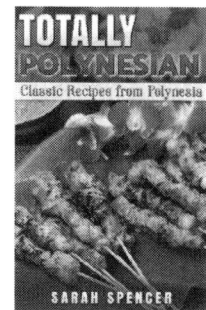

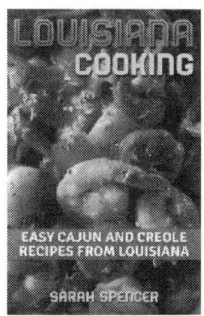
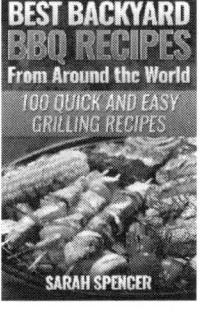
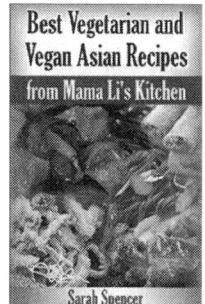

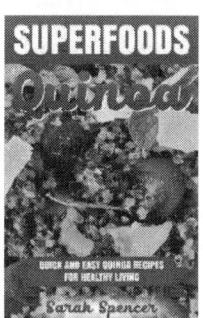

Appendix - Cooking Conversion Charts

1. Measuring Equivalent Chart

Type	Imperial	Imperial	Metric
Weight	1 dry ounce		28g
	1 pound	16 dry ounces	0.45 kg
Volume	1 teaspoon		5 ml
	1 dessert spoon	2 teaspoons	10 ml
	1 tablespoon	3 teaspoons	15 ml
	1 Australian tablespoon	4 teaspoons	20 ml
	1 fluid ounce	2 tablespoons	30 ml
	1 cup	16 tablespoons	240 ml
	1 cup	8 fluid ounces	240 ml
	1 pint	2 cups	470 ml
	1 quart	2 pints	0.95 l
	1 gallon	4 quarts	3.8 l
Length	1 inch		2.54 cm

* Numbers are rounded to the closest equivalent

2. Oven Temperature Equivalent Chart

T(°F)	T(°C)
220	100
225	110
250	120
275	140
300	150
325	160
350	180
375	190
400	200
425	220
450	230
475	250
500	260

* $T(°C) = [T(°F)-32] * 5/9$
** $T(°F) = T(°C) * 9/5 + 32$
*** Numbers are rounded to the closest equivalent

Printed in Great Britain
by Amazon